THIS JOURNAL BELONGS TO

____

Made in United States
Orlando, FL
07 May 2023

32888359R00067